AF541116

Cumulative Student Activity Record of Clinical Experience for Basic BSc Nursing Program (Log Book)

Cumulative Student Activity Record of Clinical Experience for Basic BSc Nursing Program (Log Book)

As per INC Guidelines

Second Edition

HCL Rawat
Professor and Principal
University College of Nursing
A Constituent College of
Baba Farid University of Health Sciences
Faridkot, Punjab, India

Raj Rani
Professor and Principal
College of Nursing
All India Institute of Medical Sciences
Jodhpur, Rajasthan, India

Foreword
SS Gill

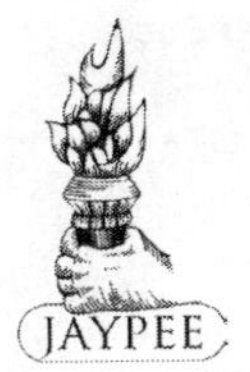

The Health Sciences Publisher
New Delhi | London | Panama

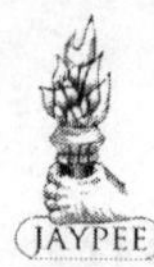

Jaypee Brothers Medical Publishers (P) Ltd

Headquarters

Jaypee Brothers Medical Publishers (P) Ltd
4838/24, Ansari Road, Daryaganj
New Delhi 110 002, India
Phone: +91-11-43574357
Fax: +91-11-43574314
Email: jaypee@jaypeebrothers.com

Overseas Offices

J.P. Medical Ltd
83 Victoria Street, London
SW1H 0HW (UK)
Phone: +44 20 3170 8910
Fax: +44 (0)20 3008 6180
Email: info@jpmedpub.com

Jaypee-Highlights Medical Publishers Inc
City of Knowledge, Bld. 235, 2nd Floor, Clayton
Panama City, Panama
Phone: +1 507-301-0496
Fax: +1 507-301-0499
Email: cservice@jphmedical.com

Jaypee Brothers Medical Publishers (P) Ltd
17/1-B Babar Road, Block-B, Shaymali
Mohammadpur, Dhaka-1207
Bangladesh
Mobile: +08801912003485
Email: jaypeedhaka@gmail.com

Jaypee Brothers Medical Publishers (P) Ltd
Bhotahity, Kathmandu, Nepal
Phone +977-9741283608
Email: kathmandu@jaypeebrothers.com

Website: www.jaypeebrothers.com
Website: www.jaypeedigital.com

Inquiries for bulk sales may be solicited at: jaypee@jaypeebrothers.com

Cumulative Student Activity Record of Clinical Experience for Basic BSc Nursing Program (Log Book)

First Edition: **2012**

Second Edition: **2017**

ISBN: 978-93-5270-011-0

Printed at Replika Press Pvt. Ltd.

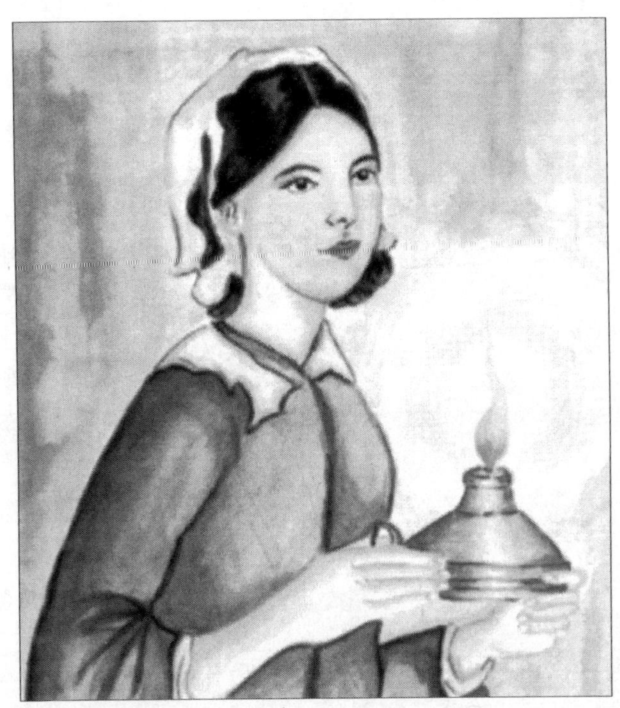

Florence Nightingale

A Lady with the Lamp

12 May 1820–13 August 1910

Nurses' Pledge

I solemnly pledge myself before God

and in the presence of this assembly,

to pass my life in purity

and to practice my profession faithfully

I will abstain from whatever is deleterious and mischievous,

and will not take or knowingly administer any harmful drug.

I will do all in my power to maintain

and elevate the standard of my profession,

and will hold in confidence

all personal matter committed to my keeping,

and all family affairs coming to my knowledge

in the practice of my calling.

With loyalty I will Endeavor

to aid the physician in his work,

and devote myself to the welfare of

those committed to my care.

Foreword

The Nursing colleges running under the state of Punjab were previously affiliated to different universities of Punjab. Since 1999, all the colleges clubbed together and now affiliated to Baba Farid University of Health Sciences, Faridkot, Punjab, India in order to bring about uniformity in course contents, teaching methods and examination evaluations system and which is based on INC, University curriculum and the recommendations of the Nursing Board of study. The faculty members of the University College of Nursing (A Constituent College of Baba Farid University of Health Sciences, Faridkot, Punjab, India) strongly felt need of developing an effective, comprehensive and cumulative clinical activity record to supplement revised curriculum to enhance clinical skills among nursing trainees. I am happy that this book is, for recording cumulative clinical experiences, prepared by Prof HCL Rawat and Prof Raj Rani with the support of faculty members of University College of Nursing as per the regulations of Indian Nursing Council and the revised curriculum of Baba Farid University of Health Sciences.

Every nursing college must recognize the importance of skillful clinical practical training and progress made by the students throughout the course. I think this record book will help in developing skills and build working confidence during the performing procedures in clinical areas. This record will provide useful information even for appointing examiners in the field of nursing. It helps in evaluation regarding the practical experience gained by individual nurse trainee during the course. I am sure that this record, which is comprehensive in its nature shall be well appreciated by the nursing students, demonstrators as well as the faculty members of Baba Farid University of Health Sciences.

Prof (Dr) SS Gill
Former Vice Chancellor
Baba Farid University of Health Sciences
Faridkot, Punjab, India

Preface to the Second Edition

Psychomotor domains, skills for performing nursing procedures are the vital components in a clinical practice which need adequate knowledge and perfection in performing skills/procedures and repeated practices. Clinical activities mentioned in this record book are minimum requirement to obtain the BSc nursing degree. The core activities of clinical experience is that students will be able to understand, comprehend and correlate the theoretical knowledge with practice and develop various skills based on scientific principles in performing number of clinical activities related to nursing.

The main purpose of this clinical activities record is to explore that the various nursing procedure skills have been demonstrated/taught by nursing faculty with expected level of satisfaction to provide quality nursing care to the individual, community, etc. independently in their future career. This record book would provide uniform learning opportunity regarding practices experienced by the student nurse under strict clinical supervision during the course.

This cumulative clinical activities record book is designed according to new syllabus approved by INC and Faculty of Nursing Sciences, Baba Farid University of Health Sciences, Faridkot, Punjab, India for BSc Nursing course.

This practical experience record book is a written document and very important for the student nurses as well as for teachers to assist the systematic learning process of the students. All the nursing procedures should be learned by following the scientific and systematic principles.

We are indeed immensely grateful to Ms Ruby Sharma of Jaypee Brothers Medical Publishers, New Delhi who urged us to embark on this venture and provided all kind of assistance and encouragement to complete this Cumulative Student Activity Record Book of Clinical Experience for BSc students.

HCL Rawat
Raj Rani

Preface to the First Edition

Psychomotor domains, skills for performing nursing procedures are the vital components in a clinical practice which need adequate knowledge and perfection in performing skills/procedures and repeated practices. Clinical activities mentioned in this record book are minimum requirement to obtain the BSc nursing degree.

The core activities of clinical experience is that students will be able to understand, comprehend and correlate the theoretical knowledge with practice and develop various skills based on scientific principles in performing number of clinical activities related to nursing.

The main purpose of this clinical activities record is to explore that the various nursing procedure skills have been demonstrated/taught by nursing faculty with expected level of satisfaction to provide quality nursing care to the individual, community, etc. independently in their future career.

This record book would provide uniform learning opportunity regarding practices experienced by the student nurse under strict clinical supervision during the course.

This cumulative clinical activities record book is designed according to new syllabus approved by INC and Faculty of Nursing Sciences, Baba Farid University of Health Sciences, Faridkot, Punjab, India for BSc Nursing course.

HCL Rawat

Student's Identification Profile

Paste passport size photograph

Name of the Student: ____________________
(In capital letters)

Father's Name: ____________________

Registration No.: ____________________

Date of Birth: ____________________

Date of Joining the Course: ____________________

Date of Completion of the Course: ____________________

Permanent Address: ____________________

____

____

____

Telephone Number ____________________ **E-mail:** ____________________

____
Signature of Student

Date

____
Signature of the Principal

Date

College Seal

General Objectives

During the clinical postings in the various areas of general specialties, the nursing students will be able to understand, comprehend and develop skills in performing the various procedures, strictly following the related scientific principles and rationales for every step adopted.

Contributory Objectives

During the clinical postings, the students will be able to:

- Correlate the theory with clinical practice.
- Acquire skills and techniques of nursing procedures in clinical settings.
- Correlate the knowledge from other disciplines while performing the steps of the procedures.
- Use systematic approach in performing the procedures.
- Assemble and check all equipment required for the procedure.
- Demonstrate skills in performing the procedures accurately based on scientific principles.
- Develop skills in assessing, planning, implementing and evaluating the nursing care in different setups, i.e. hospital and community.
- Assess the learning needs of clients, plan and implement the health education.
- Develop ability in documentation – reporting accurately and promptly.

Instructions for Proper Use of Procedure Record Book

- The purpose of maintaining a record of practical work is to ensure that the student nurse has been instructed in the various types of nursing procedures and to record whether or not she/he has performed the procedure to the satisfaction of the clinical instructor.
- The purpose of keeping the record is fulfilled only if entries are made regularly and with care. The students' record sheet should be marked every week after a discussion with the students.
- It is desirable that all procedures should be demonstrated in classroom before they are carried out in the wards/ clinical settings.
- All the procedures should be signed when the students have done it satisfactory in classroom as well as in ward by the respective clinical instructors/demonstrators. In some cases where this is not possible, the procedure is signed after return–demonstration in the demonstration room only. In such cases, the clinical instructor/demonstrator should indicate this by writing DR after his/her signature with a circle around the DR.
- No student should be permitted to do any procedure independently unless she/he has obtained a signature for that procedure.
- Procedures are to be signed after sufficient practice in the clinical areas.
- The student is expected to take responsibility for her/his own learning by:
  - Requesting the clinical instructor/demonstrator to supervise a procedure she/he needs to have signature.
  - Volunteering for experience she/he needs.
  - Taking responsibility for obtaining a signature from clinical instructor/demonstrator who has supervised the procedure, immediately following the successful completion of a procedure.
- Evaluation of students' performance should be carried out periodically.
- Students must have all the procedures signed, to be eligible for viva and practical examination for each year and should present the same to the examiners.
- Students should ensure that they get signatures from internal and external examiners after completion of practical examination every year.

Ist Year Basic BSc (Nursing)

HOURS OF INSTRUCTION

Theory: Clinical Experiences:

S. No.	Subjects	Theory (Hours)	Practical (Hours)
1	Anatomy	60	–
2	Physiology	60	–
3	Nutrition	60	–
4	Biochemistry	30	–
5	Nursing Foundations	265 + 200	450
6	Psychology	60	–
7	Microbiology	60	–
8	Introduction of Computer	45	–
9	English	60	–
Total Hours		**900**	**450**
Total Hours		**1350**	

SUBJECTS AND MARKS DISTRIBUTIONS FOR INTERNAL ASSESSMENT AND UNIVERSITY EXAMINATIONS

S. No.	Subjects	Hours	Internal Assessment	External Assessment	Total
1	Anatomy and Physiology	3	25	75	100
2	Nutrition and Biochemistry	3	25	75	100
3	Nursing Foundations	3	25	75	100
4	Microbiology	3	25	75	100
5	Psychology	3	25	75	100
6	Introductions to Computers	–	100	–	100
7	English	3	25	75	100
Practical and Viva Voce					
1	Nursing Foundations		100	100	200

Note: Introduction to computer as college level examination, by respective colleges and marks to be sent to the university.

NURSING FOUNDATIONS

S. No.	Nursing Procedures	Lab Demonstration by Demonstrator		Clinical Demonstration by Student (Verified by Demonstrator)		Remarks
		Date	Signature	Date	Signature	
1	**Preparation of Patient's Unit**					
	• Care of Patient's Unit					
	• Disinfections of the Unit					
2	**Bed Making**					
	• Unoccupied Bed					
	• Occupied Bed					
	• Operation Bed					
	• Fowler's/Cardiac Bed					
	• Amputation/Divided Bed					
	• Burns Bed					
	• Fracture Bed					
3	**Admission and Discharge**					
	• Admission					
	– New Patient Admission					
	– Transfer In					
	• Making and Maintaining Patient's Record					
	• Death Record					
	• Discharge of Patients					
	– From the Hospital					
	– Transfer Out					
	– Discharge and Counseling					
	– Abscond/Discharge against Medical Advice (DAMA)					
	• Care of Bed and Equipment after Discharge					

Contd...

Contd...

S. No.	Nursing Procedures	Lab Demonstration by Demonstrator		Clinical Demonstration by Student (Verified by Demonstrator)		Remarks
		Date	Signature	Date	Signature	
4	**Vital Signs**					
	• Temperature					
	– Oral					
	– Auxiliary					
	– Rectal					
	• Pulse					
	• Respiration					
	• Blood Pressure					
5	**Positions**					
	• Dorsal Recumbent					
	• Lateral (Rt/Lt)					
	• Prone					
	• Fowler's/Semi-Fowler's					
	• Sims					
	• Trendelenburg					
	• Lithotomy					
6	**Comfort Devices**					
	• Extra Pillows					
	• Backrest					
	• Cardiac Table					
	• Sand Bags					
	• Bed Cradle					
	• Trochanter Rolls					
	• Cotton Rings and Hand Rolls					

Contd...

Contd...

S. No.	Nursing Procedures	Lab Demonstration by Demonstrator		Clinical Demonstration by Student (Verified by Demonstrator)		Remarks
		Date	Signature	Date	Signature	
	• Air Rings/Air Cushion					
	• Water/ Air Mattress					
7	**Safety Measures and Infections Control**					
	• Handwashing					
	– Medical					
	– Surgical					
	• Practical Universal Precautions					
	– Use of Masks					
	– Use of Gloves					
	– Use of Gowns					
	• Disposal of Wastes					
	• Side Rails					
	• Protective Padding					
	• Restraints					
	• Foot end Elevator					
8	**Hygienic Needs**					
	• Bed Bath					
	• Assisted Bath					
	• Back Care					
	• Oral Hygiene					
	• Care of Nails, Hands and Feet					
	• Bed Shampoo and Hair					
	• Wash					
	• Pediculosis Treatment					
	• Eye/Ear/Nose Care					

Contd...

Contd...

S. No.	Nursing Procedures	Lab Demonstration by Demonstrator		Clinical Demonstration by Student (Verified by Demonstrator)		Remarks
		Date	Signature	Date	Signature	
9	**Care of Hospital Articles**					
	• Rubber Articles					
	– Air Cushions					
	– Rubber Mackintosh					
	– Hot Water Bottle					
	– Ice Cap					
	– Rubber Gloves					
	– Rubber Tubes					
	• Enamel Articles					
	– Bedpan					
	– Urinals					
	– Sputum Mug					
	• Glass Articles					
	– Syringes					
	– Test Tube					
	– Ounce Glass					
	• Needles					
	• Sharp Instruments					
	• Stainless Steel Articles					
	• Linen					
	• Mattress and Pillows					
10	**Preparation and Sterilization**					
	• Physical					
	• Boiling					

Contd...

Contd...

S. No.	Nursing Procedures	Lab Demonstration by Demonstrator		Clinical Demonstration by Student (Verified by Demonstrator)		Remarks
		Date	Signature	Date	Signature	
	• Autoclaving					
	• Flaming					
	• Hot Air Oven					
	• Chemical					
	• Mechanical					
	• Preparation of Antimicrobial Solutions					
11	**Nutritional Needs**					
	• Serving Normal Diet					
	• Therapeutic/Modified Diet					
	• Bland Diet					
	• Salt Restricted					
	• Diabetic Diet (Low Calorie)					
	• High Protein Diet					
	• Hepatic Comma Diet					
	• Renal Diet					
12	**Elimination Needs**					
	• Assisting Patients in Urinary Elimination					
	• Giving and Removing Urinal					
	• Giving and Removing Bedpan					
	• Enema					
	• Suppository					
	• Bowel Wash					
	• Insertion of Flatus Tube					
	• Perineal Care					

Contd...

Contd...

S. No.	Nursing Procedures	Lab Demonstration by Demonstrator		Clinical Demonstration by Student (Verified by Demonstrator)		Remarks
		Date	Signature	Date	Signature	
	• Condom Drainage					
	• Catheterization					
	• Care of Urinary Drainage					
13	**Collection of Observation of Specimen**					
	• Urine					
	• Routine					
	• Culture					
	• 24 Hours					
	• Stool/Feces					
	– Routine					
	– Culture					
	• Blood					
	– Routine					
	– Culture					
	– Peripheral Smear					
	• Vomitus					
	• Throat Swab					
	• Urine Test					
	– Reaction					
	– Specific Gravity					
	– Albumin					
	– Sugar					
	– Acetone					
	– Bile Pigments and Salts					

Contd...

Contd...

S. No.	Nursing Procedures	Lab Demonstration by Demonstrator		Clinical Demonstration by Student (Verified by Demonstrator)		Remarks
		Date	Signature	Date	Signature	
14	**Nursing Process**					
	• Assessment					
	– History Taking					
	– Physical Examination					
	• Nursing Diagnosis					
	• Planning					
	• Implementation					
	• Evaluation					
15	**Therapeutic Measures**					
	• Medications					
	• Calculation and Measuring Doses					
	• Administration of Medications in Different Forms and Routes					
	• Oral Medication					
	• Parenteral Medication					
	– Intradermal Injection					
	– Subcutaneous Injection					
	– Intramuscular Injection					
	• Assisting in Intravenous Infusion					
	• Assisting in Blood Transfusion					
	• Administration of Oxygen by Different Methods					
	• Steam Inhalation					
	• Nebulization					
	• Instillation of Drops: Eye, Ear, Nose					
	• Oral, Nasal Suctioning					

Contd...

Contd...

S. No.	Nursing Procedures	Lab Demonstration by Demonstrator		Clinical Demonstration by Student (Verified by Demonstrator)		Remarks
		Date	Signature	Date	Signature	
	• Pre and Postoperative Care					
	• Hot and Cold Application					
	• Hot Water Bag					
	• Sitz Bath					
	• Cold Compress					
	• Ice Cap					
	• Tepid Sponge/Cold Sponge					
16	**Body Mechanics/Alignment Mobility and Exercise**					
	• Changing Position of Helpless Patient					
	• Lifting and Handling of Bedridden Patients					
	• Transferring Bed to Wheelchair, Trolley and Back					
	• Active/Passive Exercises					
	• Chest Physiotherapy					
	• Helping the Patient with use of Crutches and Walker					
	• Care of Postural Drainage					
17	**First Aid**					
	• First Aid for fracture					
	– Application of slings					
	– Application of splints					
	• Shock and Burns					
	• Unconsciousness					
	• Poisoning, Bites and Stings					
	• First Aid in Hemorrhage and Other Emergency					
	– Pressure bandage					
	– Cold application					

Contd...

Contd...

S. No.	Nursing Procedures	Lab Demonstration by Demonstrator		Clinical Demonstration by Student (Verified by Demonstrator)		Remarks
		Date	Signature	Date	Signature	
	– Cardiopulmonary Resuscitation (CPR)					
	– Preparation of First Aid Kit					
18	**Bandaging**					
	• Simple Spiral					
	• Reverse Spiral					
	• Figure of Eight					
	• Spica					
	• Head/Cap line					
	• Eye, Ear, Jaw					
	• Finger, Elbow, Knee					
	• Stump, Various Knots					
	• Use of Triangular Bandage					
	• Use of Binders					
	• Dressing of Wound					
19	**Management of Patients with Common Problems**					
	• Care of Patients with Pyrexia					
	• Care of Patients with Dyspnea					
	• Care of Patient with Unconsciousness					
	• Care of Patients with Paralysis					
	• Care of Patients with Plaster Cast					
	• Care of Patients with Traction					
	• Care of Dying and Dead Body					
20	**Health Education**					
	• Individual					
	• Group					

NURSING CARE PLANS

S. No.	Date	Disease Condition	Signature
1			
2			
3			
4			
5			

Signature of Class Coordinator

Signature of Principal

Practical Examination
Nursing Foundations

Signature of Internal Examiner

Date:

Signature of External Examiner

Date:

Signature of Internal Examiner

Date:

Signature of External Examiner

Date:

IInd Year Basic BSc (Nursing)

HOURS OF INSTRUCTION

Theory: Clinical Experiences:

S. No.	Subjects	Theory (Hours)	Practical (Hours)
1	Sociology	60	–
2	Pharmacology	45	–
3	Pathology	30	–
4	Genetics	15	–
5	Medical Surgical Nursing I (Adult Including Geriatrics)	210	720
6	Community Health Nursing I	90	135
7	Communication and Educational Technology	60 + 30	–
Total Hours		**540**	**855**
Total Hours		**1395**	

SUBJECTS AND MARKS DISTRIBUTIONS FOR INTERNAL ASSESSMENT AND UNIVERSITY EXAMINATIONS

S. No.	Subjects	Hours	Internal Assessment	External Assessment	Total
1	Sociology	3	25	75	100
2	Medical Surgical Nursing I	3	25	75	100
3	Pharmacology, Pathology and Genetics	3	25	75	100
4	Community Health Nursing I	3	25	75	100
5	Communications and Educational Technology	3	25	75	100
Practical and Viva Voce					
1	Medical Surgical Nursing I		100	100	200

MEDICAL SURGICAL NURSING I (ADULT INCLUDING GERIATRICS)

S. No.	Nursing Procedures	Lab Demonstration By Demonstrator		Clinical Demonstration by Student (Verified by Demonstrator)		Remarks
		Date	Signature	Date	Signature	
1	**Preoperative Preparation**					
	• Preoperative preparation of skin					
	• Preoperative medication					
2	**Postoperative Care**					
	• Setting of Postoperative Unit					
	• Postoperative Care					
	• Recovery Room					
	• Ward					
	• Surgical Dressing					
	• Removal of Sutures					
3	**Operation Theater Technique**					
	• General Preparation of Operation Theater					
	– Preparation and Packing of Articles for Surgery					
	– Disinfection/Carbolization, Fumigations of the Operation Theater					
	– Surgical Scrubbing					
	– Gown and Gloves					
	– Setting up of Trolley for Different Surgeries					
	• Packing of Drums					
	– Instruments					
	– Linen					
	– Gloves					
	• Endotracheal					
	– Intubation and Suctioning					
	– Extubation					

Contd...

Contd...

S. No.	Nursing Procedures	Lab Demonstration By Demonstrator		Clinical Demonstration by Student (Verified by Demonstrator)		Remarks
		Date	Signature	Date	Signature	
	• Preoperative Skin Preparation					
	• Assessment and Assisting in Anesthesia					
	• Assisting in Major Surgery					
	1					
	2					
	3					
	4					
	5					
	• Assisting in Minor Surgery					
	1					
	2					
	3					
	4					
	5					
4	**Observation of Specific Diagnostic and Therapeutic Procedures**					
	• Vascular System					
	– Intravenous (IV) Cannulation					
	– Doppler Studies					
	– ECG Recording and Interpretation					
	– Cardiac Catheterization					
	– Invasive/Non-invasive Procedures					
	– Intra-aortic Balloon Pump (IABP)					
	– Cardiopulmonary Resuscitation (CPR)					

Contd...

Contd...

S. No.	Nursing Procedures	Lab Demonstration By Demonstrator		Clinical Demonstration by Student (Verified by Demonstrator)		Remarks
		Date	Signature	Date	Signature	
	• Genitourinary System					
	– Catheterization					
	– Plain					
	– Indwelling/Foley					
	– Condom Drainage					
	– Bladder Irrigation					
	– Cystoscopy					
	– Intravenous Pyelogram (IVP)					
	– Kidney, Ureter, Bladder (KUB)					
	– Assisting in Peritoneal Dialysis					
	– Assisting in Hemodialysis					
	– Assisting in Renal Biopsy					
	• Chemical Regulation					
	– Fasting Blood Sugar (FBS)					
	– Postprandial Blood Sugar (PPBS)					
	– Glucose Tolerance Test (GTT)					
	– Administration of Insulin					
	– Thyroid Function Test – T3, T4, TSH					
	• Gastrointestinal System					
	– Barium Meal					
	– Barium Enema					
	– Proctoscopy					
	– Endoscopy					
	– Cholecystography					
	– Esophagogastroduodenoscopy (EGD)					
	– Ostomy Care					

Contd...

Contd...

S. No.	Nursing Procedures	Lab Demonstration By Demonstrator		Clinical Demonstration by Student (Verified by Demonstrator)		Remarks
		Date	Signature	Date	Signature	
	– Liver Biopsy					
	– Live Function Tests (LFTs)					
	– Insertion and Removal of Nasogastric Tube					
	– Endoscopic Retrograde Cholangiopancreatography (ERCP)					
	• Musculoskeletal System					
	– Physiotherapy/Crutch Maneuver Technique					
	– Preparation, Assisting Application and Removal of Plaster Cast					
	– Assisting in Skin Traction					
	– Assisting in Skeletal Traction					
	– Preparation of Patient for Bone Surgery					
	– Stump Care					
	– Application and Removal of Prosthesis					
	– Rehabilitation of Patient with Prosthesis					
	• Skin and Communicable Diseases					
	– Practice Medical and Surgical Asepsis					
	– Practice Standard Safety Measures					
	– Counseling HIV Positive Patient					
	– Health Teaching for Prevention of Infectious Diseases					
	• Cardiovascular System					
	– Physical Assessment of Cardiac Patient					
	– Monitoring of Cardiac Patient					

Contd...

Contd...

S. No.	Nursing Procedures	Lab Demonstration By Demonstrator		Clinical Demonstration by Student (Verified by Demonstrator)		Remarks
		Date	Signature	Date	Signature	
	– Administering Cardiac Drugs					
	– Assisting in Cardiopulmonary Resuscitation					
	• Respiratory System					
	– Oxygen Therapy by Different Methods					
	– Nebulization					
	– Chest Physiotherapy					
	– Perform and Assist in Therapeutic Procedure					
	• Nutrition					
	– Tube Feeding/Nasogastric Feeding					
	– Gastrostomy/Jejunostomy Feeding					
	– Intake Output Chart					
	– Parenteral Feeding					
5	**Specific Therapeutic Procedures**					
	• Assisting in ECG (Electrocardiogram)					
	• Assisting in Venous Puncture					
	• Assisting in Abdominal Paracentesis					
	• Assisting in Thoracentesis					
	• Assisting in Lumbar Puncture					
	• Assisting in Gastric Lavage					
	• Assisting in Sternal Puncture					
6	**Pharmacology**					
	• Preparation of Emergency Drug Trolley					
	• Inotropic Agents					
	• Emergency Cardiac Drugs					
	• Preparation and Maintenance of IV Fluids					

NURSING CARE PLANS

S. No.	Date	Disease Condition	Signature
1			
2			
3			
4			
5			

COMMUNITY HEALTH NURSING I

S. No.	Nursing Procedures	Lab Demonstration by Demonstrator		Clinical Demonstration by Student (Verified by Demonstrator)		Remarks
		Date	Signature	Date	Signature	
1	Preparation and Maintenance of Family Records					
2	Conduct Community Survey and Report					
3	Conduct Family Health Survey and Report					
4	Demonstrate bag Technique					
5	Comprehensive Family Study					
6	Preparation and Use of Audio-Visual (AV) Aids					
7	Participate in Family Welfare Programs					
8	Participate in Primary Health Care (PHC) Clinics					
9	Assist in Immunization Programs					
10	Motivation for Family Planning					
11	Monitoring Growth and Development					
12	Treatment or Minor Aliments					
13	Home Care of TB Patient					
14	Care of Elderly at Home					
15	Health Teaching/Information Education Communication (IEC)/Behavior Change Communication (BCC) Activities					
	• Individual					
	• Group					

Contd...

Contd...

S. No.	Nursing Procedures	Lab Demonstration by Demonstrator		Clinical Demonstration by Student (Verified by Demonstrator)		Remarks
		Date	Signature	Date	Signature	
16	Assessment of Nutritional Status in Various Age Group					
17	Nutritional Education					
18	Visits					
	• Community Health Center (CHC)					
	• Primary Health Center (PHC)					
	• Subcenter (SC)					
	• Aanganwadi Center					
	• Postpartum Center					
	• Milk Plant/Dairy					
	• Water Purification/Sewage Plant					

FAMILY CARE STUDY

S. No.	Name: Head of the Family	House No.	Urban/Village	Date	Signature of Demonstrator
1					
2					
3					
4					
5					

HEALTH TEACHING

S. No.	Name of the Topic	Area/Group	Date of Teaching	Signature of Demonstrator
1				
2				
3				
4				
5				

Signature of Class Coordinator

Signature of Principal

PRACTICAL EXAMINATION

Medical Surgical Nursing I
(Adult Including Geriatrics)

Signature of Internal Examiner
Date:

Signature of External Examiner
Date:

Signature of Internal Examiner
Date:

Signature of External Examiner
Date:

IIIrd Year Basic BSc (Nursing)

HOURS OF INSTRUCTION

Theory: Clinical Experiences:

S. No.	Subjects	Theory (Hours)	Practical (Hours)
1	Medical Surgical Nursing II (Adult including Geriatrics)	120	270
2	Child Health Nursing	90	270
3	Mental Health Nursing	90	270
4	Midwifery and Obstetrical Nursing	90	180
	Total Hours	**390**	**990**
	Total Hours	**1380**	

SUBJECTS AND MARKS DISTRIBUTIONS FOR INTERNAL ASSESSMENT AND UNIVERSITY EXAMINATIONS

S. No.	Subjects	Hours	Internal Assessment	External Assessment	Total
1	Medical Surgical Nursing II	3	25	75	100
2	Child Health Nursing	3	25	75	100
3	Mental Health Nursing	3	25	75	100
Practical and Viva Voce					
1	Medical Surgical Nursing II		50	50	100
2	Child Health Nursing		50	50	100
3	Mental Health Nursing		50	50	100

MEDICAL SURGICAL NURSING II (ADULT INCLUDING GERIATRICS)

S. No.	Nursing Procedures	Lab Demonstration by Demonstrator		Clinical Demonstration by Student (Verified by Demonstrator)		Remarks
		Date	Signature	Date	Signature	
1	**Eye and Ear, Nose and Throat (ENT) Ward/Unit**					
	• Instillation of Drops/Ointment					
	– Eye					
	– Ear					
	– Nose					
	• Perform Eye examination					
	• Eye Irrigation					
	• Care of Patient with Eye Surgery					
	1					
	2					
	3					
	4					
	5					
	• Perform ENT examinations					
	• Ear Irrigation					
	• Throat Swab culture					
	• Tracheotomy Care					
	• Assist in Removal of Foreign Bodies					
2	**Neurology and Neurosurgery Ward/Unit**					
	• Neurological Assessment of Patient					
	• Glasgow Coma Scale					
	• Care of Patient with Cervical Traction					

Contd...

Contd...

S. No.	Nursing Procedures	Lab Demonstration by Demonstrator		Clinical Demonstration by Student (Verified by Demonstrator)		Remarks
		Date	Signature	Date	Signature	
	• Care of Patient with Paralysis of Limbs					
	• Neurovascular assessment					
	• Preparing Patient for Electroencephalogram (EEG)					
	• Preparing Patient for Magnetic Resonance Imaging (MRI)					
3	**Burns and Scalds**					
	• Assessment of Burn's Patient					
	• Assessment of Area and Degree of Burns					
	• Prepare and Calculate Fluid Requirement of Burn Patient					
	• Administration of Fluid and Electrolytes					
	• Assist in Burn's Dressing					
	• Preparing for Reconstructive Surgery and Donor Area					
	• Perform Exercise for Burn Patient					
	• Rehabilitation of Burn Patient					
4	**Oncology Ward/Unit**					
	• Preparation and Assist in Biopsies					
	• Assist in Radiotherapy					
	• Assist in Chemotherapy					
	• Care of Patient with Chemotherapy					
	• Assist in Bone Marrow Aspiration					

Contd...

Contd...

S. No.	Nursing Procedures	Lab Demonstration by Demonstrator		Clinical Demonstration by Student (Verified by Demonstrator)		Remarks
		Date	Signature	Date	Signature	
5	**Gynecology Ward/Unit**					
	• Assist in Gynecological Examination					
	• Assist in Diagnostics Procedures					
	• Pap Smear					
	• Perform Breast Self-Examination (BSE)					
6	**Critical Care/Unit**					
	• Monitoring of Patient in Critical Care Unit					
	• Assisting in Endotracheal Intubations					
	• Suctioning					
	– Endotracheal					
	– Tracheostomy					
	– Oral/Nasal					
	• Assist with Arterial Puncture					
	• Monitoring and Maintaining Central Venous Pressure (CVP) Line					
	• Demonstrate Use of					
	– Mechanical Ventilators					
	– Cardiac Monitors					
	– Pulse Oximetry					
	– Defibrillator					
	– Bag and Mask					
	– Infusion Pump					

Contd...

Contd...

S. No.	Nursing Procedures	Lab Demonstration by Demonstrator		Clinical Demonstration by Student (Verified by Demonstrator)		Remarks
		Date	Signature	Date	Signature	
	• Total Parenteral Therapy					
	• Chest Physiotherapy					
	• Perform Active and Passive Exercises					
	• Cardiopulmonary Resuscitation: Basic Life Support/Advanced Life Support (BLS/ALS)					
	• Care of Patient on Ventilator					
7	**Casualty and Emergency**					
	• Receiving Patient in Emergency Unit					
	• Assessment of Patient on Emergency Trolley					
	• Triage Applications					
	• Assist in Disaster Situations					
	• Assist in Legal Procedures in Casualty					
	• Assist in Examination of Patients in Casualty					
	• Oxygen Administration					
	• Drug Therapy/Inotropes in Emergency					

NURSING CARE PLANS

S. No.	Date	Disease Condition	Signature
1			
2			
3			
4			
5			

CHILD HEALTH NURSING

S. No.	Nursing Procedures	Lab Demonstration by Demonstrator		Clinical Demonstration by Student (Verified by Demonstrator)		Remarks
		Date	Signature	Date	Signature	
1	**Admission/Discharge of Children**					
2	**History Taking**					
3	**Physical Assessment/Physical Examination**					
4	**Growth and development monitoring**					
5	**Calculation of Medicines Doses**					
6	**Administration of Medication**					
	• Oral					
	• Intramuscular					
	• Intravenous					
7	**Preparation of Oral Rehydration Solution (ORS)**					
8	**Calculation of IV Fluid Required for Children**					
9	**Fluid Preparation (N/5, N/4, N/3, N/2) in 5% or 10% Dextrose**					
10	**Methods of Oxygen Administration in Children**					
11	**Collection of Specimens**					
	• Urine (Male and Female)					
	• Blood					
	• Throat Swabs					
12	**Assist in Breastfeeding**					
	• Exclusive Breastfeeding					
	• Paladie and Katori Spoon					

Contd...

Contd...

S. No.	Nursing Procedures	Lab Demonstration by Demonstrator		Clinical Demonstration by Student (Verified by Demonstrator)		Remarks
		Date	Signature	Date	Signature	
	• Nasogastric Feeding					
	• Gastrostomy Feeding					
	• Jejunostomy Feeding					
13	**Care of Ostomies**					
	• Colostomy Stoma Care					
	• Colostomy Irrigation					
14	**Care of Child In/On**					
	• Incubator					
	• Ventilator					
	• Overhead Warmer					
	• Phototherapy					
15	**Use of Restraints**					
	• Mummy Restraints					
	• Elbow Restraints					
	• Clove-Hitch Restraints					
16	**Assist In Special Therapeutic Procedures**					
	• Lumbar Puncture					
	• Resuscitation					
	• Phototherapy					
	• Exchange Transfusion					
	• Therapeutic Play					

Contd...

Contd...

S. No.	Nursing Procedures	Lab Demonstration by Demonstrator		Clinical Demonstration by Student (Verified by Demonstrator)		Remarks
		Date	Signature	Date	Signature	
17	**Planning Special Diet for Children**					
	• Nephrotic Syndrome					
	• Protein Energy Malnutrition					
	• Hepatic Encephalopathy					
	• Renal Failure					
	• Diabetic diet					
18	**Care during Pediatric Emergencies**					
	• Asphyxia					
	• Convulsion					
	• Head Injury					
	• Foreign Body Aspiration					
19	**Participation in Immunization Health Teaching/IEC/BCC Activities**					
	• Individual					
	• Group					
20	**Visits**					
	• Center for Physically, Mentally, Challenged Certified School					
	• SOS Village					
	• Other agencies related to child health service					

NURSING CARE PLANS

S. No.	Date	Disease Condition	Signature
1			
2			
3			
4			
5			

MENTAL HEALTH NURSING

S. No.	Nursing Procedures	Lab Demonstration by Demonstrator		Clinical Demonstration by Student (Verified by Demonstrator)		Remarks
		Date	Signature	Date	Signature	
1	**Admission/Discharge of the Psychiatric Patient**					
2	**Mental Status Examination (MSE)**					
3	**Process Recording**					
4	**Nursing Care of Patient with**					
	• Psychotic Disorder					
	• Neurotic Disorder					
	• Organic Conditions					
	• Character Disorder					
	• Substance Abuse					
5	**Assist in Specific Therapies**					
	• Electroconvulsive Therapy					
	• Psychotherapy					
	• Occupational Therapy					
	• Behavioral Therapy					
	• Recreational Therapy, Play Therapy					
	• Milieu Therapy, De-Addiction Therapy					
6	**Administration of Psychotherapeutic Drugs**					
7	**Community Psychiatry**					
	• Conduct Case Work/Study					
	• Identify Person with Mental Health Bless					
	• Assist in Mental Health Camps					

NURSING CARE PLANS

S. No.	Date	Disease Condition	Signature
1			
2			
3			
4			
5			

MIDWIFERY AND OBSTETRICAL NURSING

S. No.	Nursing Procedures	Lab Demonstration by Demonstrator		Clinical Demonstration by Student (Verified by Demonstrator)		Remarks
		Date	Signature	Date	Signature	
1	**Prenatal Care**					
	• Prenatal Assessment					
	• Prenatal Care					
	• Preparation for Non Stress Test (NST) and Ultrasound					
2	**Intranatal Care**					
	• Setting up of Newborn Resuscitation Unit					
	• Perineal Preparation for Labor					
	• Partogram					
	• Per Vaginal (PV) Examination					
	• Normal Delivery					
	• Episiotomy and Suturing					
	• Apgar Scoring					
	• Resuscitation of Newborn					
3	**Postnatal Care**					
	• Postnatal Assessment					
	• Postnatal Care					
	• Perineal Light					

Contd...

Contd...

S. No.	Nursing Procedures	Lab Demonstration by Demonstrator		Clinical Demonstration by Student (Verified by Demonstrator)		Remarks
		Date	Signature	Date	Signature	
	• Care of Breast					
	• Assisting with Breastfeeding					
4	**Newborn Care**					
	• Assessment of Newborn					
	• Care of Normal Newborn					
	• Care of High-risk Newborn					
5	**Requirements**					
	• Conducts Antenatal (30)					
	• Provides Antenatal Care (5)					
	• Witness Normal Deliveries (20)					
	• Conduct Normal Deliveries (Hospital and Home)					
	• Episiotomy and Suturing (2)					
	• Provide Postnatal Care					
	– Hospitalized (20)					
	– Home					

Note: Number in brackets indicate minimum number of procedures to be witness or done.

NURSING CARE PLANS

S. No.	Date	Disease Condition	Signature
1			
2			
3			
4			
5			

PRACTICAL EXAMINATION

Medical Surgical Nursing II

(Adult Including Geriatrics)

Signature of Internal Examiner	Signature of External Examiner
Date:	Date:
Signature of Internal Examiner	Signature of External Examiner
Date:	Date:

Child Health Nursing

Signature of Internal Examiner	Signature of External Examiner
Date:	Date:
Signature of Internal Examiner	Signature of External Examiner
Date:	Date:

Mental Health Nursing

Signature of Internal Examiner	Signature of External Examiner
Date:	Date:
Signature of Internal Examiner	Signature of External Examiner
Date:	Date:

IVth Year Basic BSc (Nursing)

HOURS OF INSTRUCTION

Theory:

Clinical Experiences:

S. No.	Subjects	Theory (Hours)	Practical (Hours)
1	Midwifery and Obstetrical Nursing	–	180
2	Community Health Nursing II	90	135
3	Nursing Research and Statistics	45	–
4	Management of Nursing Services and Education	60 + 30	–
	Total Hours	**225**	**315**
	Total Hours	**540**	

SUBJECTS AND MARKS DISTRIBUTIONS FOR INTERNAL ASSESSMENT AND UNIVERSITY EXAMINATIONS

S. No.	Subjects	Hours	Internal Assessment	External Assessment	Total
1	Midwifery and Obstetrical Nursing	3	25	75	100
2	Community Health Nursing II	3	25	75	100
3	Nursing Research and Statistics		25	75	100
4	Management of Nursing Service and Education	3	25	75	100
Practical and Viva Voce					
1	Midwifery and Obstetrical Nursing		50	50	100
2	Community Health Nursing II		50	50	100

MIDWIFERY AND OBSTETRICAL NURSING

S. No.	Nursing Procedures	Lab Demonstration by Demonstrator		Clinical Demonstration by Student (Verified by Demonstrator)		Remarks
		Date	Signature	Date	Signature	
1	**Prenatal Care**					
	• Antenatal History Taking					
	• Physical Examination of Antenatal Mother					
	• Set-up of Antenatal and Postnatal Clinic					
	• Genetic Counseling and Planned parenthood					
	• Set-up of Obstetric ICU (Eclampsia Unit)					
2	**Care of High-Risk Antenatal Mother**					
	• Preeclampsia					
	• Eclampsia					
	• Placenta Previa					
	• Abruptio Placenta					
	• Gestational Diabetes					
	• Cardiac Diseases					
	• Rh Incompatibility					
	• Preterm Contraction					
	• HIV/AIDS/Viral Infections					

Contd...

Contd...

S. No.	Nursing Procedures	Lab Demonstration by Demonstrator		Clinical Demonstration by Student (Verified by Demonstrator)		Remarks
		Date	Signature	Date	Signature	
3	**Intranatal Care**					
	• Induction of Labor					
	• Assist/Witness Obstetric Procedures					
	– Forceps Delivery					
	– Vacuum Extraction					
	• Assist/Witness Breach Delivery					
	• Assist/Witness Multifetal					
	• Delivery					
	• Assist/Witness Cesarean Section					
	• Assist D and E, D and C					
	• Assist and Perform Episiotomies and Suturing					
4	**Postnatal Care**					
	• Care of High-risk Postnatal Mothers					
	• Perineal Care					
	– Resuscitation of Newborn Baby					
	– Lactation Management					
	– Baby Bath					

Contd...

Contd...

S. No.	Nursing Procedures	Lab Demonstration by Demonstrator		Clinical Demonstration by Student (Verified by Demonstrator)		Remarks
		Date	Signature	Date	Signature	
	– Kangaroo Mother Care (KMC)					
	– Postnatal Exercises					
5	**Family Welfare**					
	• Motivation of Planned Parenthood					
	• Assist/Perform IUCD Insertion					
	• Assist/Observe Tubectomy					
	• Assist/Observe Vasectomy					
6	**Requirements**					
	• Witness Normal Deliveries (10)					
	• Assist in Abnormal Deliveries (5)					
	• Motivation of Planned Parenthood (2)					
	• Attend Antenatal and Parenthood					
	• Provide Care to High-risk Antenatal Mothers					
	• Provide Care to High-risk Neonates (5)					
	• Provide Care to High-risk Postnatal Mother (5)					
	• Witness/Assist Cesarean Section (5)					

Note: Number in brackets indicate minimum number of procedures to be witness or done.

ANTENATAL CARE PLAN/CARE STUDY

S. No.	Date	Disease Condition	Signature
1			
2			
3			
4			
5			

POSTNATAL CARE PLAN/CARE STUDY

S. No.	Date	Disease Condition	Signature
1			
2			
3			
4			
5			

NEONATAL CARE PLAN/CARE STUDY

S. No.	Date	Disease Condition	Signature
1			
2			
3			
4			
5			

COMMUNITY HEALTH NURSING II

S. No.	Nursing Procedures	Lab Demonstration by Demonstrator		Clinical Demonstration by Student (Verified by Demonstrator)		Remarks
		Date	Signature	Date	Signature	
1	**Community Health Survey**					
2	**Comprehensive Family Health Care**					
3	**Organizing and Assisting in**					
	• Antenatal and Postnatal Clinic					
	• Immunization					
	• Family Welfare Activities					
	• School Health Programs					
	• Health Camps					
4	**Project Work and Presentation of Reports**					
5	**Records**					
	• Family Folder					
	• Individual					
6	**Health Education/IEC/BCC**					
	• Urban					
	• Rural					
7	**Participate in National Health Programs**					
8	**Counsel and Teach Individual, Family, Community about HIV, TB, DM, etc.**					
9	**Home Visits**					
10	**Bag Technique**					
11	**Supervise Health Workers**					
12	**Visits**					
	• School					
	• Industry					
	• Community Health Nursing					
	• Red Cross					
	• Professional Bodies Like Trained Nurses Association of India (TNAI), Indian Nursing Council (INC), Punjab Nursing Registration Council (PNRC)					
	• Epidemic Diseases Hospital					

COMPREHENSIVE FAMILY HEALTH CARE

S. No.	Date	Disease Condition	Signature
1			
2			
3			
4			
5			

MANAGEMENT OF NURSING SERVICES AND EDUCATION

S. No.	Nursing Procedures	Lab Demonstration by Demonstrator		Clinical Demonstration by Student (Verified by Demonstrator)		Remarks
		Date	Signature	Date	Signature	
1	**Supervision**					
	• Students					
	• Staff					
	• Ward Aides					
2	**Preparation of Duty Roster**					
3	**Preparation of Ward Records**					
4	**Preparation of Work Assignment**					
	• Students					
	• Staff					
	• Ward Aides					
5	**Reporting**					
	• Oral					
	– Morning					
	– Evening					
	– Night					
	• Written					
	– Day					
	– Night					
6	**Inventory**					
	• Drugs					
	• Articles					
7	**Maintain Census**					
8	**Conduct Nursing Round**					
9	**Preparation of Teaching Aids**					
	• Preparation of Lesson Plan					
	• Charts					

Contd...

Contd...

S. No.	Nursing Procedures	Lab Demonstration by Demonstrator		Clinical Demonstration by Student (Verified by Demonstrator)		Remarks
		Date	Signature	Date	Signature	
	• Posters					
	• Flash Cards					
	• Transparencies					
	• Power Point					
10	**Preparation of Master Rotation Plan**					
11	**Conduct Clinical Teaching**					
	1					
	2					
12	**Conduct Clinical Teaching**					
	1					
	2					
13	**Preparation of Job Description for Different Categories**					
	• Principal					
	• Nursing Superintendent					
	• Clinical Instructor/Demonstrator					
	• Ward Sister/Head Nurse					
	• Staff Nurse					
14	**Preparation of Evaluation Tool to Assess the Patient Care**					
15	**Educational Tour to Various Institutions and Professional Bodies and Submit the Report**					

Signature of Class Coordinator

Signature of Principal

PRACTICAL EXAMINATION

Midwifery and Obstetrical Nursing

Signature of Internal Examiner	Signature of External Examiner
Date:	Date:
Signature of Internal Examiner	Signature of External Examiner
Date:	Date:

Community Health Nursing II

Signature of Internal Examiner	Signature of External Examiner
Date:	Date:
Signature of Internal Examiner	Signature of External Examiner
Date:	Date:

RESEARCH PROJECT

Note: Group of students should have options to select the research project in their area of interest in the beginning of the internship in consultation with their respective supervisor.

Title of the Research Project: ______________________________

____

____

____

____

____

Date of Submission of Report: ______________________________

Date of Presentations: ______________________________

____
Name and Signature of Supervisor

____
Signature of Principal

BASIC IMPORTANT FORMULAS

- **Conversion Formulas**
  - Conversion of Fahrenheit scale to Celsius scale

    $C = (F - 32) \times \frac{5}{9}$
  - Conversion of Celsius scale to Fahrenheit scale

    $F = (C \times \frac{9}{5}) + 32$
  - Inches to centimeter

    I inch = 2.54 cm

    1 cm = 0.39 inch
  - Minim to milliliter (ml)

    1 minims = 0.06 ml

    1 ml = 16 minims
  - Equivalent imperial and metric quantities

1 grain	=	65 milligrams
1 ounce	=	28 grams
1 pound	=	453 grams
1 tea spoon	=	3 tea spoon = 15 ml
1 tea cup	=	150–180 ml
1 standard glass	=	240–250 ml
1 ounce	=	30 ml
1 pound	=	16 ounces
1 kg	=	2.2 pounds
1 drop	=	1/20 ml or 0.05 ml
1 pint	=	500 ml

- **Important Formulas**
  - Body mass index (BMI)

    $$BMI = \frac{\text{Weight in kg}}{\text{Height in (meter)}^2}$$
  - Estimation of child's dose calculation
    - According to body surface area

      $$\text{Child's dose} = \frac{\text{Child's body surface area}}{\text{Adult's body surface area}} \times \text{Adult dose}$$

      Young's Formula, According to Age

      $$\text{Child's dose} = \frac{\text{Age of Child}}{\text{Age} + 12} \times \text{Adult dose}$$
    - Clark's Formula, According to body weight

      $$\text{Child's dose} = \frac{\text{Weight of children (16 pound)}}{150} \times \text{Adult dose}$$

- Calculating flow rate

$$\text{Drop/Minute} = \frac{\text{Total volume to infused}}{\text{Time in minute}} \times \text{Drop factor}$$

Drop Factor
Micro drip set
60 drops = 1 ml
Macro drip set
16 drops = 1 ml

- Infusion time calculation

$$\text{Infusion time} = \frac{\text{Total volume to infusion}}{\text{ml per hour being infused}}$$

– Expected date of delivery
  EDD = Date of LMP + 9 month + 7 days
– Percentage of malnutrition

$$\text{Malnutrition} = \frac{\text{Actual weight}}{\text{Expected weight}} \times 100$$

– Formula for calculating expected weight
  - For Age (1 month to 12 months)

$$\text{Weight} = \frac{\text{Age in months} + 9}{2}$$

  - For Age (1 – 6 years)
    Weight = (Age in years × 2) + 8
  - For Age (6–12 years)

$$\text{Weight} = \frac{(\text{Age in years} \times 9) - 5}{2}$$

  - Normal birth weight of Indian Newborn 2.5–3 kg
  - Birth weight doubles by the age of 5–6 months
  - Birth weights triples by the age of 1 years.
  - Four times by 2 years, five time by 3 years and 10 times by 10 years.
– Calculation of Height
  - At birth = about 45 to 55 cm
  - At 1 year of age = about 75 cm
  - Birth height double by 4–4 ½ years
  - At 1–12 years of age
    Height = (Age in years × 6) + 77 cm
    or
    Height = (Age in years × 6) + 66 cm
– Intelligence quotient calculation formula

$$\text{Intelligence quotient} = \frac{\text{Mental age}}{\text{Chronological age}} \times 100 \text{ or IQ} = \frac{\text{MA}}{\text{CA}} \times 100$$

FLUID REQUIREMENT FOR NEWBORN BABY AND PEDIATRIC CLIENTS

Formulas for calculating fluid requirement for pediatric clients.

Upto 10 kg body weight 100 ml/kg/day

11–20 kg body weight 50 ml/kg/day

21 kg onwards 20 ml/kg/day

For Example: A baby weighing 9.5 kg required fluid according to body weight

9.5 × 100–950 ml/24 hours

12 kg body weight

10 × 100 = 1000

2 × 50 = 100 = 1100 ml/24 hours

22 kg body weight

10 × 100 = 1000

10 × 50 = 500

2 × 20 = 40 = 1540 ml/24 hours

Types of fluids commonly used in pediatric area:

N/5 in 5% or 10% Dextrose

N/4 in 5% or 10% Dextrose

N/3 in 5% or 10% Dextrose

N/2 in 5% or 10% Dextrose

Dextrose 10% and Ringer Lactate

USEFUL NORMAL LABORATORY VALUES

Blood/Serum

Bleeding Time (BT)	1 to 3 minutes
Clotting Time (CT)	3 to 10 minutes
Erythrocyte Sedimentation Rate (ESR)	Male less than 20–30 mm/hr
Platelets count	2,00,000—4,50,000/cumm
Hemoglobin	Female 12–16 gm%, Male 14–16 gm%
WBC Count	5000–10,000, cumm (7500 cumm)
Neutrophils%	40–75% (60%)
Esinophils %	1–6%
Basophils %	0–1%
Lymphocytes %	20–45% (30%)
Monocytes %	2–10%
Reticulocytes %	0.2%
Blood sugar (fasting)	60–100 mg/dl
Blood sugar PP/Random	120–150 mg/dl
Blood urea	10–40 mg/dl
Serum Creatinine	0.5–1.4 mg/dl
Serum cholesterol	130–250 mg/dl
Serum Bilirubin (Total)	0.2–1.0 mg/dl
Serum Bilirubin (Direct)	0.0–0.2 mg/dl
Serum Bilirubin (Indirect)	0.2–0.8 mg/dl
Uric Acid	2.5–7.0 mg/dl
Calcium	8.8–10.8 mg/dl
Sodium	135–155 meq/Ltr
Phosphorus	1.5–6.8 mg/dl
Chloride	90–107 meq/dl
Total protein	6.3–8.3 gm/dl
Albumin	3.5–5.5 gm/dl
SGOT	4 to 40 u/l
SGPT	5 to 45 u/l
Triglycerides	40–160 mg/dl
Total Lipids	400–700 mg/dl
pH Value	7.35–7.45 (Adult)

URINE OUTPUT AT DIFFERENT AGES

S. No.	Age	Normal Urine output (ml/24 hr)
1	Newborn	250
2	2 months	450
3	1 year	500
4	2 years	550
5	4 years	650
6	7 years	750
7	11 years	1100
8	14 years	1200
9	Adult	1500

CLINICAL POSTING FOR THE BASIC BSC NURSING STUDENTS

Month	First Year	Second Year	Third Year	Fourth Year	Remarks
August					
September					
October					
November					
December					
January					
February					
March					
April					
May					
June					
July					

Signature of the Class Coordinator

Date:

Signature of the Principal